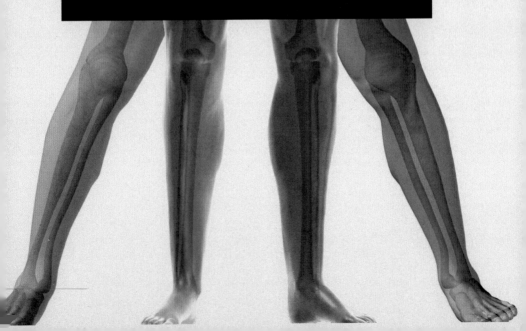

THE
PRIVATE
SQUARE

Volume 1: Penises

TABITHA KATZ

The Private Square
Volume 1: Penises
All Rights Reserved.
Copyright © 2013 Tabitha Katz
v10.0 Second Printing

CreateSpace, a DBA of On-Demand Publishing, LLC.
ISBN-13: 978-1511691734
ISBN-10: 1511691735
http://www.the privatesquare.com

PRINTED IN THE UNITED STATES OF AMERICA

Table of Contents

Foreword

Everyone wonders about his or her body. Everyone worries about how his or her body stacks up in comparison to the array of bodies around them. What is "*in*" regarding body types at this point in time? What is normal, attractive, alluring, or impressive? What matters? The author of *The Private Square* has provided the real, unedited truth about our bodies. In her four part series, Tabitha Katz has courageously given the reader proof and prose about the penises, breasts, vulvas and buttocks of many people without bias or retouching. *The Private Square* masters the art of show, don't tell, while giving honest representations of the body parts people worry the most about. There is no norm; there is no right way to look.

This author's exceptional work, *The Private Square* series, answers many questions and qualms about bodies. The media today exposes the public to highly sexualized versions of humans; it is no wonder that the common perception of how we "should" look is skewed. Does size matter? No, because we often forget that one size does not really fit all. We only need to care about the size we have and the size that would fit with each of us best; we must disregard any standard we feel held to in concern to how large or slight we are. Consider while reading this work that you are a woman who is built very small. What size partner would fit you best, most comfortably, with ease? In this innovative work, Ms. Katz affords us the opportunity, privately, to decide for ourselves without pressure or bias what we really think about all of these sizes, shapes, and colors. *The Private Square* encourages regarding our bodies as a gift. Ah, the beauty of self-esteem – we are beautiful and we are not alone.

Despite numerous conversations, curiosities, and delusions of grandeur about sexual body parts, it can be difficult to find answers. The author of *The Private Square* has unveiled those truths in her series.

I have been a behaviorist in private practice for forty years. Over the years, hundreds of male and female clients have come to me carrying stress and insecurity regarding their penises, breasts, vulvas and buttocks. And while my practice is intimate, I can hardly say: "show me and we'll talk!" However, now I can say: "read *The Private Square* and we'll talk." There is great pressure from the social arena about how we "should" look. Tabitha Katz has taken a serious and gutsy approach to honestly demonstrate a large sampling of how we *actually* look. It eases the mind to see in living color that we all have differences and we are all normal! This author has provided the critical vehicle for us to look, know, and accept that our bodies are the same as countless others.

Louise F. Burnham, M.A., B.M.C.

Praise

To Louise for her enthusiasm for my project and steadfast belief that I could succeed with this series.

To my husband for taking a step back and viewing life with different eyes; and for standing by me through the production of this series. These books would never have materialized if not for his support. It took trust and courage for him to watch me drive off to take intimate photographs of strangers. He acted as my technical support; and he patiently handled my interruptions of his work to "Google" the colorful and unfamiliar terminology my clientele used. He encouraged me whole-heartedly.

To my daughters... look no further!

I love you.
TK

Introduction

As the mother of three daughters, I wondered for years what I would tell them when they asked me what a penis looked like. If you don't have a brother in the house and Dad wants to keep his privates private, there is a good chance a house full of girls won't see one until they are children playing doctor, adolescents playing Truth or Dare, or teens/young adults becoming intimate.

My youngest, as a preschooler, first registered that boys were different from girls when she shared a bathroom with her male cousins at a fire station pancake breakfast. She turned to her aunt and me, pointed, and asked, "What's that?" I explained what a penis was, and she then commented "So it just hangs there and sticks out?" Touché.

My older daughters' awareness of the penis piqued in the seventh grade when they studied the reproductive system in science class. At that age there were a lot of giggles and furtive looks around the classroom. The boys' reaction to the instruction of sexual organs was to strut their stuff like peacocks. They reclined in their desk chairs, got the girls' attention, and then pointed to the swell of an erection in their pants. During my daughters' teen years, there were even more examples of this kind of nonchalant behavior. I was astounded by how casually their generation seemed to view sexuality.

Unlike my children, it wasn't until well into my adult years that my women friends and I had discussions about penises. To the age-old question: "Does size matter?" we always concluded that fit, sensitivity to your mate, and sexual prowess mattered more than size. As you will see within these pages, penises are as unique as people. They come in all shapes, sizes, colors and hang in a multitude of ways.

It is my hope that *The Private Square: Penises* will unveil the mystery of the male's most prized body part and be a means by which men can see how normal they are. Bodies are amazing – no two penises are alike. There is truly something for everyone. *The Private Square* is a learning experience for our youth that will make them wiser, healthier, and more realistic adolescents. Positive body image is a vital factor in gaining and maintaining self-esteem. This book lays a foundation for teens and adults to be more accepting of their body, their sexuality, and themselves.

The research for *The Private Square: Penises* was conducted in a culturally diverse, major metropolitan area of the United States. Finding subjects was a unique challenge. Though I have scores of friends, acquaintances, and business associates, there were few with whom I had the relationship to ask if they would model for me semi-nude. When I did gather the courage to do so, the initial response from my late-stage Baby Boomer friends was disbelief and embarrassment.

I explained the pictures were for a photojournalism project I was embarking on. I suggested that keeping their shirt on so they would not be nude; or perhaps wear sunglasses or a low hat as a means to mask their audience, me, from their personal stage. Though my male friends understood the darkened theatre analogy, their answer was still a resounding "no." That said, as men they were fully supportive of my endeavor and asked for a signed copy upon publication!

At this point I needed to solicit strangers. Thinking that younger men would be less inhibited about their bodies, I printed colorful flyers soliciting models for a chance to make some quick money by participating in an "Educational Anatomical Photo Shoot." I proceeded to walk through multiple college and university campuses, gyms, and a few nightclubs, posting my notice on bulletin boards, in cafeterias, fraternity houses, and the walls of men's rooms. My biggest risk was posting a similar notice on Craigslist under the Talent Gigs section.

Though I was renting space in a photo studio located in a professional artists building, being a woman alone with a naked man has inherent risk. In addition, satisfying my supportive but understandably concerned husband about my safety during the "research" portion of the project was another challenge I needed to overcome. So I contacted my daughter's karate teacher, whose full-time job was teaching mixed martial arts at a local community college. He shared with me some names of his adult students who were interested in being hired as security during my photo shoots. These black belts could disarm, restrain, harm, and generally provide me with protection should the need arise.

After years of pondering the idea of a book of penises and a few weeks of planning, I had equipment, studio space, protection, and interested models.

And thus my research began…

A Dirty Ditty

The use of slang, pornography, and eroticism can both mask personal feelings about our bodies and lighten what at times is an awkward personal subject. People's discomfort or concerns with their bodies often influences a separate, but equally important part of our lives - personal sexuality. A light-hearted approach to dealing with body parts and inherent sexual desires is good for some laughs but does not make people feel better about their bodies. The dirty ditty and partial list of what surely is hundreds of synonyms that follow exemplify this notion.

Whether you are somewhat dissatisfied with your penis, breasts, vulva or buttocks, or harbor a more serious negativity, these very personal feelings can damage self-esteem and inhibit intimate relationships or sexual enjoyment. The Private Square series attempts to counter the damage from societal pressures of measuring up to media-propagated physical perfection by showing you what real people, like you and me, look like - in an honest and unaltered way.

The Private Square

Please... please, touch me there
Right in my private square
Grab my ass and pull me close
Rub your girls along my post
Take my shaft and make me moan
Kiss and lick my quiver bone
Guide my one-eyed wonder worm
In your pussy 'til we both squirm
Ride me 'til you tingle through
Then I'll explode inside of you

What's In A Name?

For men, the penis represents courage, toughness, strength, sexual prowess and virility - it is their machismo. It can be a symbol of power, used as a weapon or a means to share the utmost intimacy. Most would agree that the penis is the most personified organ of the human body. Some people give special names to the penis, whilst slang terms are prolific worldwide:

Phallus • Rod • Tool • Quiver Bone • Dick • Meat
Junk • Prick • Cock • Shaft • Dong • Worm • Boner
Woody • Mr. Big • Winkie • Johnson • Chubby
Beaver Basher • One-Eyed Wonder Worm • Peter
Divining Rod • Love Muscle • Sausage • Pickle • Pole
Knob • Stiffy • Tinker • Pecker • Wiener • PeePee
Schlong • Cyclops • Shmuck • Joystick • Baby-Maker
Anaconda • Special Offer • Hard-on • John Thomas
Hose Monster • Wang Doodle • Trouser Snake
Beaver Cleaver • Pump • Unit • Package • Doodle
Boomerang • Member • Doinker • Wankie • Love Stick
Wick • Boomerang • Putz • Magic Stick • Rod
One-Eyed Monster • Man's Best Friend • Pinocchio
The Dicktator • Love Shaft • Mr. Happy • Love Muscle
Pleasure Pump • Heat-Seeking Moisture-Missile

Finding Penis Models

Sample Ads

Wanted: adult men of any age and type as life models for paid professional, anonymous, educational photo shoot. No experience necessary - $40.

Looking for everyday, ordinary, real men to model for educational anatomy project. No faces or full body pictures taken. All photos are anonymous. Payment $40 for individual photo shoot.

Will pay $40 to take anonymous photos of your sexual body parts. No faces or full body pictures taken. Must be 18 or older. Appointments or walk-ins welcome.

Need adults 18 & older for anatomical photography project. The pay is $40 for a 10-minute, anonymous, individual session to take pix of private body parts. Release and receipt must be signed. Studio hours by appointment. Walk-ins welcome.

Seeking a widely diverse population of adults (18 or over) for an educational, anatomical, anonymous photo shoot. Young adults must show proof of age.

Responses

"Cool. I am a nice, polite, respectful gentleman and would be honored to have you take photos of my penis and balls. I am also comfortable posing with an erection."

"I am interested in your ad on craigslist.org for, 'Real Men' commercials. Thank you for letting me know if there are any appointments available."

"I'm currently a 32 year-old Spanish male seeking different opportunities; I'd like to inquire any information on making an appointment and any other information required from myself. I can see the artistic value of nudity and would love to take a part on this job."

"I'm willing to have a photo taken of my private area."

"I did a photo shoot with U a few days ago... I'm bearded & tattooed. Would U consider me again with another male if I can find one... if I not I totally understand."

"I'm a 45 year-old Latino. I'm willing to takes pictures no problem as long as my face is not posted."

"Interested in hearing more about this project. 27 year-old African American photographer, would like to be in front of the camera."

"I might not be ur type" sent a full body nude photo of himself lying on his back with arms above his head, eyes closed and penis resting on his thigh.

"To whom it may concern, if you still require additional life models, I am interested. Please send details."

"Are you a female photographer? If so I would be honored to pose nude for you for your project."

"Hi I am a 22 year-old guy looking to let you take anonymous photos of my sexual body parts. I can probably make it there from 5 to 6pm. I am 6'4" and about 240, tall and chubby. Please let me know if this will work for you."

Demographics

The Models

BY RACE	BY DEMOGRAPHICS
18% African American	43% Twenties
6% Asian	25% Thirties
58% Caucasian	8% Forties
14% Hispanic	13% Fifties
1% Indian	10% Sixties
3% Multiracial	1% Seventies

Circumcised Or Not?

BY RACE	BY AGE
72% African American	70% Twenties
50% Asian	68% Thirties
79% Caucasian	88% Forties
57% Hispanic	69% Fifties
0% Indian	90% Sixties
50% Multiracial	100% Seventies

71% of the male subjects herein are circumcised.

The Penis

The penis is one of two external organs of the male sexual/ reproductive system. It has three parts: the root, which attaches to the abdomen, the body (a.k.a. shaft), and the glans penis, which is the cone-shaped end (a.k.a. head). The opening of the urethra (the tube that transports semen and urine) is at the tip of the glans penis.

The body of the penis consists of three internal chambers. These chambers are made up of a sponge-like erectile tissue – this tissue contains thousands of large caverns that fill with blood when the man is sexually aroused. As the penis fills with blood, it becomes rigid and erect to enable penetration during sexual intercourse. The skin of the penis is loose and elastic to accommodate changes in penis size during an erection.

Semen, which contains sperm (the male reproductive cells), is expelled through the end of the penis when the man reaches sexual climax (orgasm).

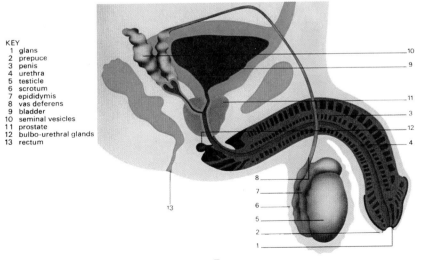

KEY
1 glans
2 prepuce
3 penis
4 urethra
5 testicle
6 scrotum
7 epididymis
8 vas deferens
9 bladder
10 seminal vesicles
11 prostate
12 bulbo-urethral glands
13 rectum

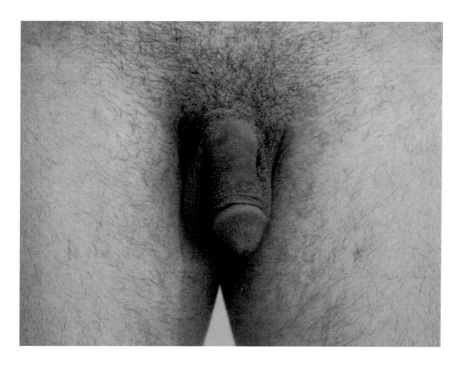

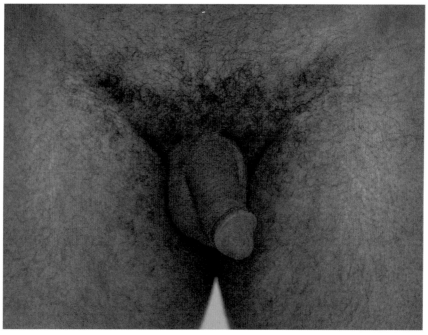

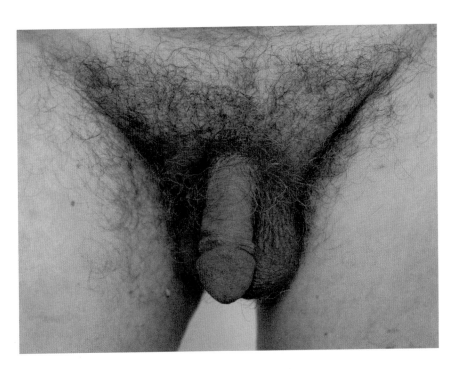

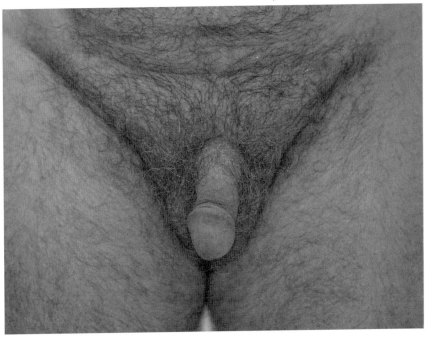

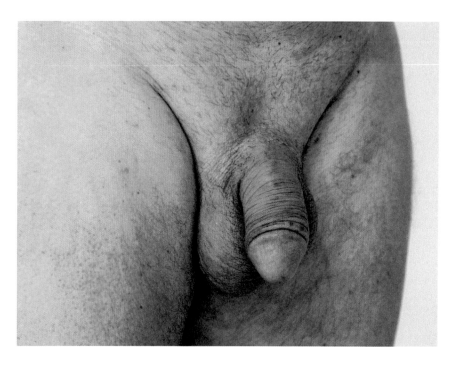

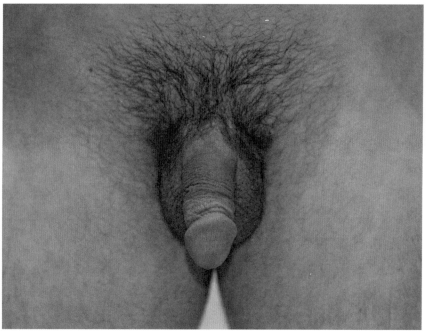

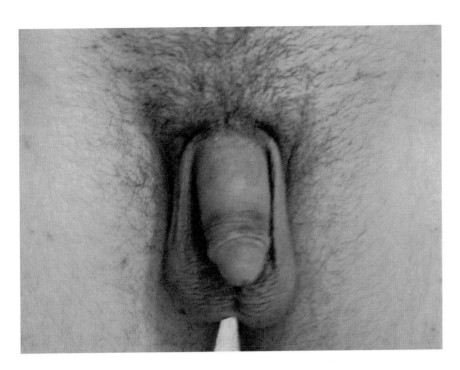

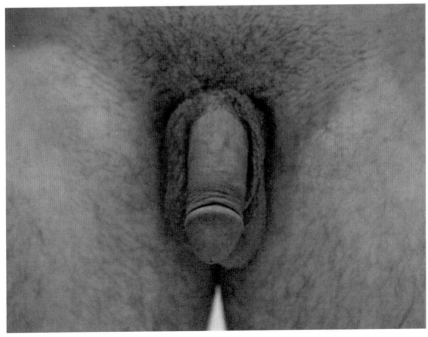

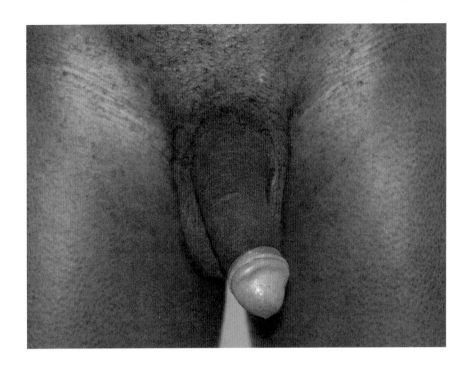

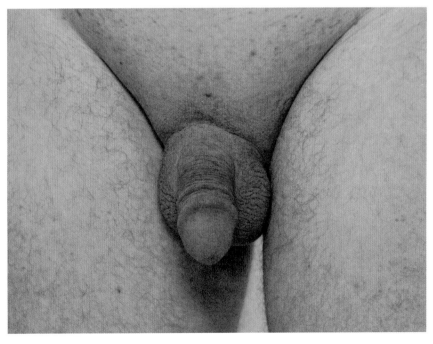

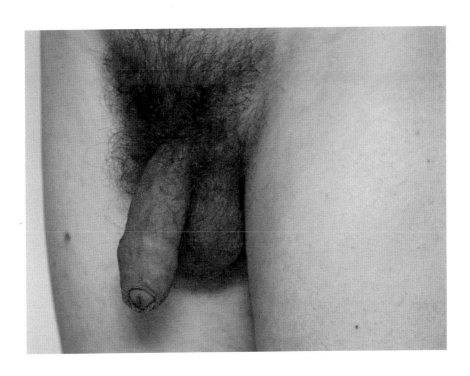

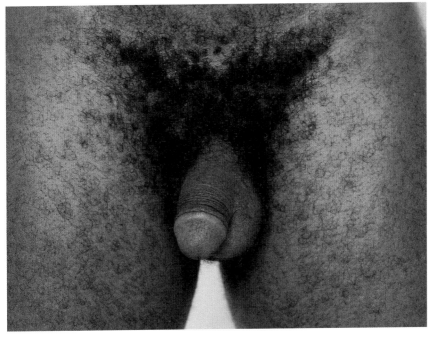

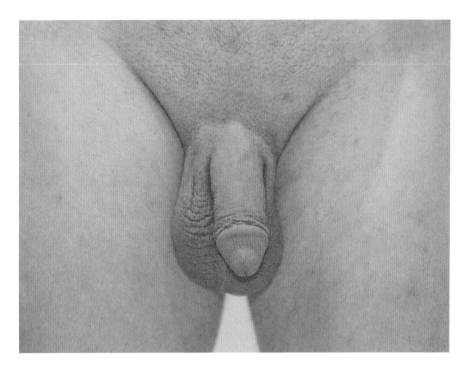

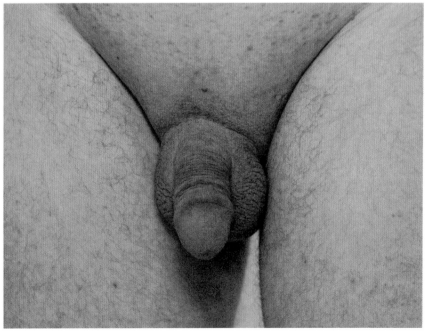

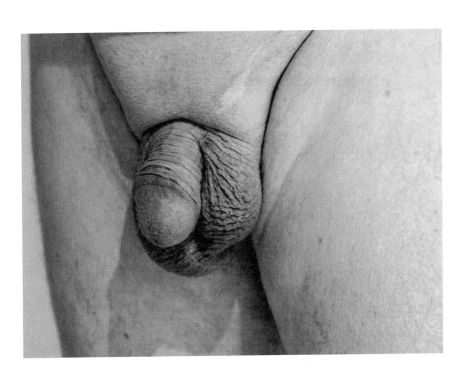

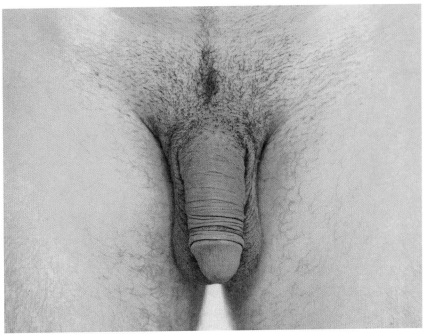

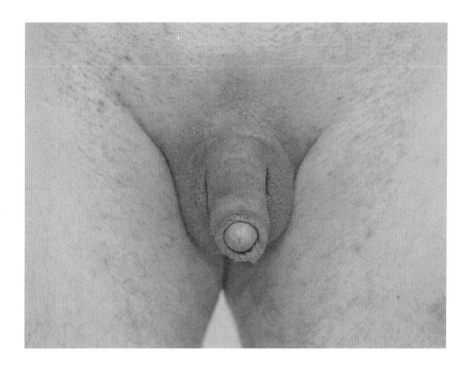

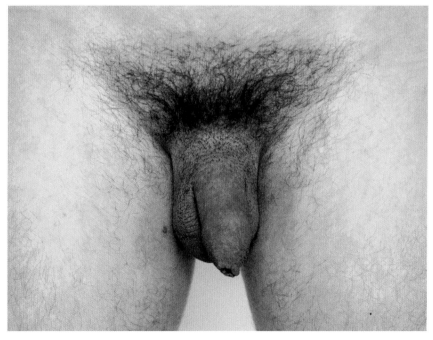

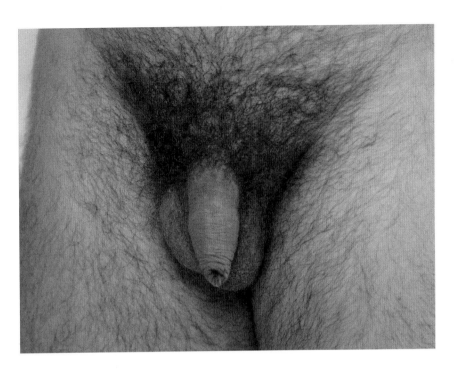

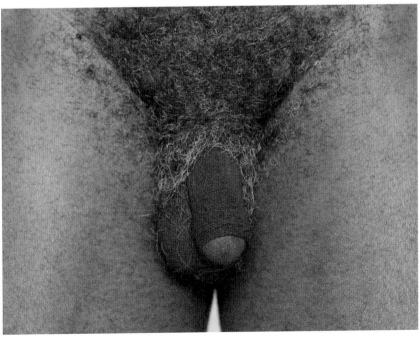

The Men: Exposed

My first client wandered in on a cold, gray, drizzly day wearing a trench coat. He was a longhaired, down-on-his-luck, 60ish, former photographer and hobbyist poet referred to me by the studio landlord. He spoke in a subdued voice, asked me about my project and removed his coat. Fortunately, he took me up on my offer to use the private (un)dressing room allowing me a chance to take a breath before snapping photos of the first adult penis, other than my husband's, that I had seen "live" in 21 years.

The second gentleman who walked into my studio, also in his 60s, claimed to be a sax-playing part-time model and former physicist. He had prolific white hair atop his head but was shaved in his southern hemisphere, a first for me. Also curious was that it appeared his testicles were undescended or even missing, as his scrotum was full and flush against his groin.

There were construction workers doing tenant improvements in the building. One dropped by, a bit skeptical about exactly what I was doing, but posed for me nonetheless. Later that day, another worker came by; then a couple more, and another. I think all of them took home some extra cash and stories from this particular subcontracting job!

A sweatshirt-hooded young man swaggered in wearing some of the baggiest saggy jeans I had ever seen. Seriously, the waistband was near his knees. How he could walk without losing his pants or tripping was beyond me. I couldn't tell what he looked like or what his body might be like at all. A large, blue eye-shadowed, pink-blushed, brightly lipsticked, bleach-blonde in skin tight animal print leggings and a bright faux fur-lined bomber jacket who looked old enough to be his mother was his escort... Hmmm? Undressed, he was built like Adonis. What?!?

Later a young man in his 20s came in with his girlfriend. She was warm and encouraging, but he was clearly uncomfortable. I assured him the photo shoot was completely voluntary. His response was to tell me he was embarrassed because he had genital warts and asked if I could photograph the "healthy side" of his penis." I did.

One of my favorite clients was a man who felt awkward because he was not circumcised. That led to a discussion about the data I collected on circumcision and customs he learned while travel-ing in the US and Europe. Ultimately we had a successful photo shoot. A few days later, he sent me an email thanking me for the opportunity to participate in my project. He then wrote that he had spoken to his girlfriend about me and how I was "a very laid-back and attractive woman." Further, he wrote that he and his girlfriend are "both bisexual and polyamorous." They were wondering if perhaps I was polyamorous and open to a ménage à trois or, if I had a partner to join us, in a ménage à quatre. I would be able to come to their place and take any amount of photographs I desired. My immediate response was to send my regrets – "I am very flattered but no thank you" – to the client AND to call my husband to find out whether he had ever heard the term "polyamorous!"

One of the most touching interactions I had was with an 18 year-old girl and her slightly older boyfriend. She was dressed in cute jeans, a colorful camisole, high-heeled boots, and a flowery purse. When I began to talk to them, I swiftly ascertained that my client was transgender/transsexual, and the soft-spoken girl was actually male by birth. She was very shy and clearly embarrassed by her "boy parts" and asked if she could keep them squeezed between and behind her legs for the pictures. I photographed her with and without her male parts showing.

Another favorite client was a 60 year-old Latino man who sauntered in dressed in very metropolitan attire. He was the definition of debonair. I am not sure what he had more pride in – his classy wife, his physique, or the realistic, red-inked kiss tattoo next to his well-groomed landing strip.

One 21 year-old gay man came in with a coed who was a friend of my family. He was quite nervous but determined to participate in my project. So we talked and talked and talked… he went into the dressing room and came out in a robe. We talked and talked and talked some more. Finally, we did a run-through with him in the robe. He said he couldn't really see me because I was hidden behind my camera lens, affixed to a bulky tripod. He took a deep breath, disrobed, and posed for me. Afterwards he told me it had been "the most emancipating" thing he had done in his entire life!

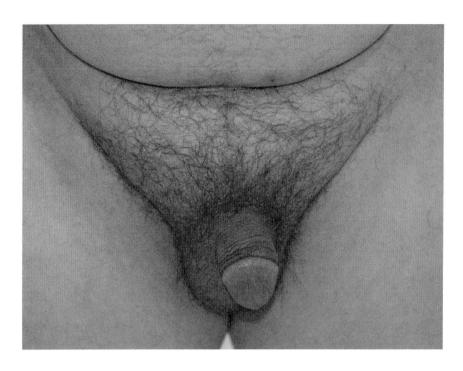

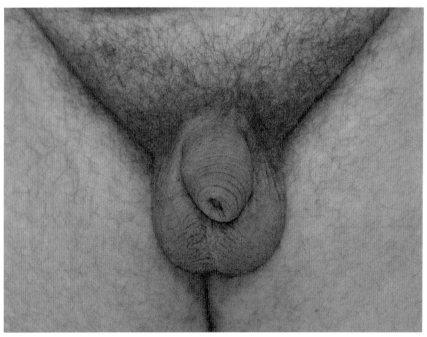

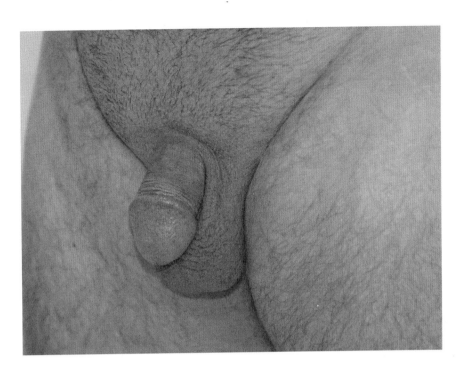

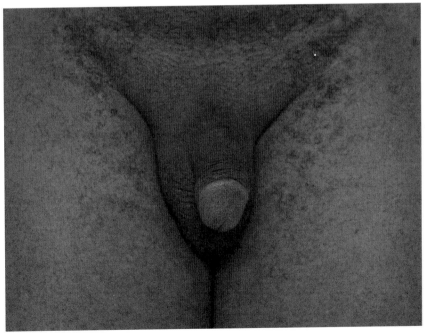

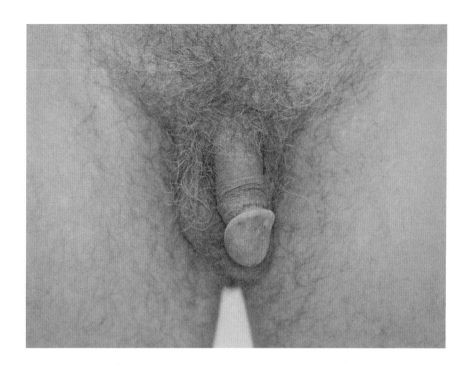

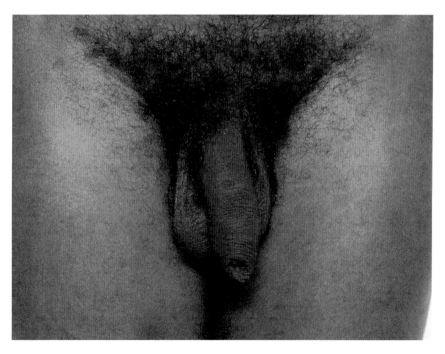

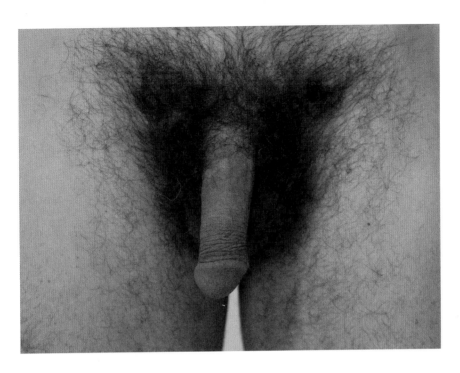

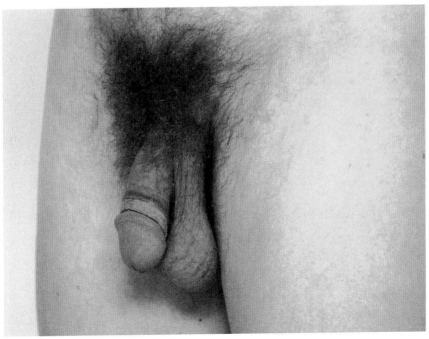

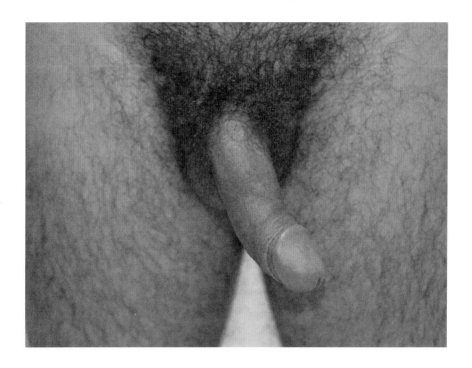

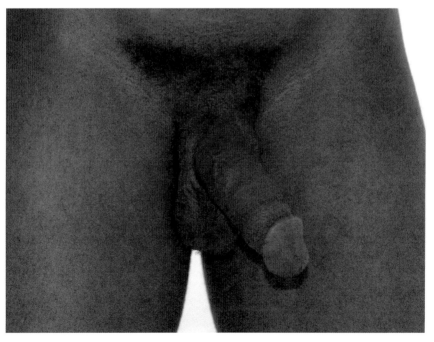

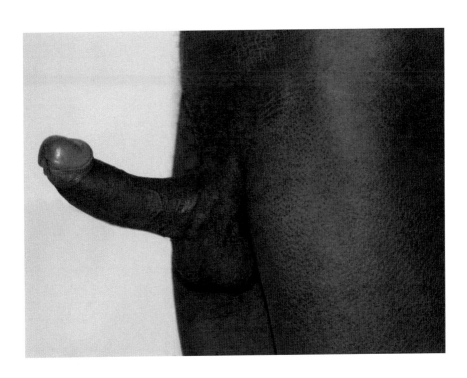

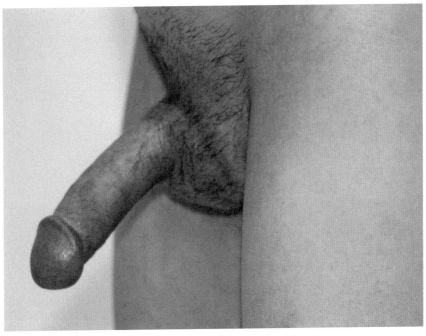

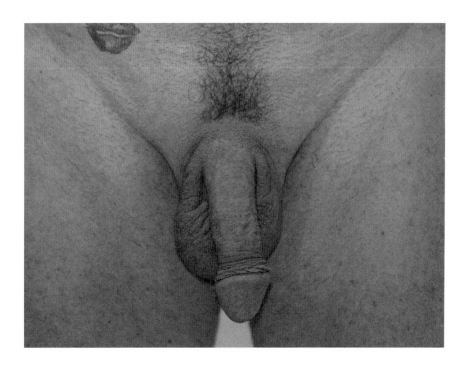

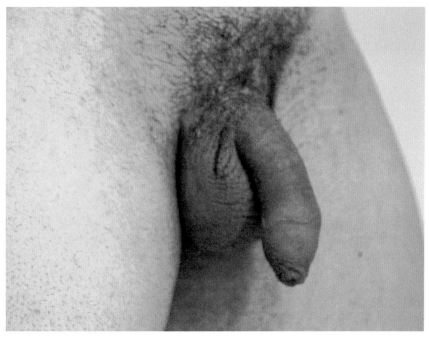

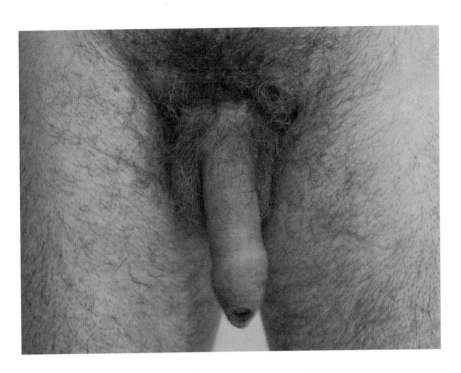

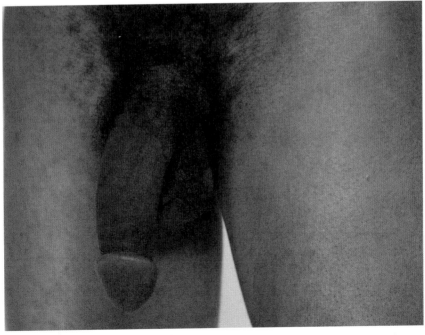

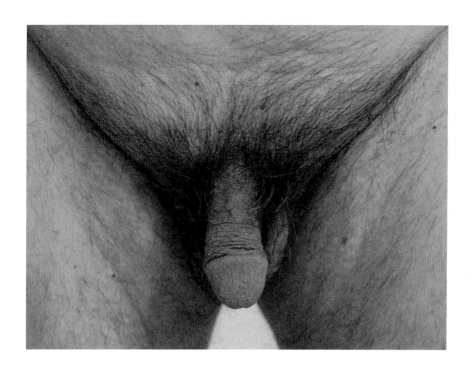

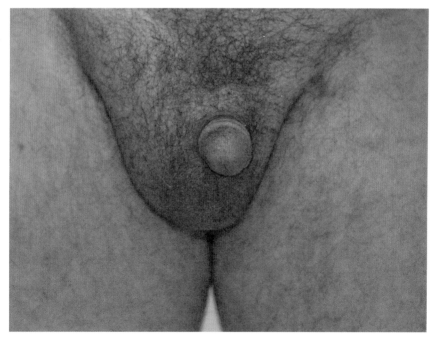

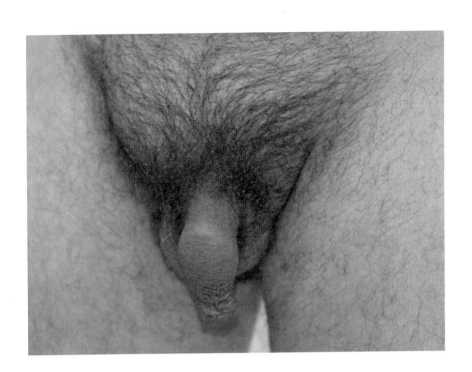

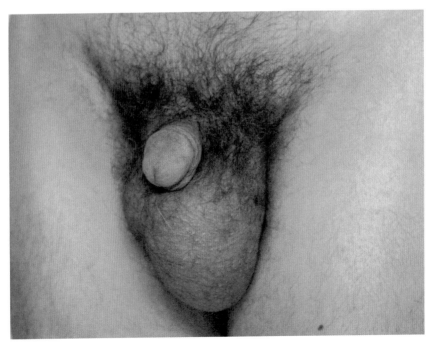

Hernias

The men pictured in the top row of the previous pages (30-31) are both afflicted withan inguinal (iNG-gwə-nəl) hernia. Inguinal refers to the groin. Notice the bulge in their right groin – the area where their torso meets the top of their leg. An inguinal hernia occurs when part of your inner fat or small intestine bulges through an anatomical passageway that is over-large, has been weakened, or is torn. There are two types of inguinal hernias.

An **indirect inguinal hernia** is a congenital condition caused by the way males develop in utero. In a male fetus, the spermatic cord and both testicles normally descend through the inguinal canal into the scrotum, the sac that holds the testicles. Some-times the entrance of the inguinal canal at the inguinal ring does not close as it should just after birth, leaving a weakness in the abdominal wall. Fat or part of the small intestine slides through the weakness into the inguinal canal, causing a hernia. Indirect hernias are the most common type of inguinal hernia.

Direct inguinal hernias are caused by connective tissue degeneration of the abdominal muscles, which causes weakening of the muscles during the adult years. Direct inguinal hernias occur predominantly in males. A direct hernia develops gradually because of continuous stress on the muscles. One or more of the following factors can cause pressure on the abdominal muscles and may worsen the hernia: sudden twists, pulls, muscle strains, lifting heavy objects, straining on the toilet because of constipation, weight gain, and/or chronic coughing.

Indirect and direct inguinal hernias usually slide back and forth spontaneously through the inguinal canal and can often be moved back into the abdomen with gentle massage. If enough time passes without repair, the hernia can worsen.[1]

[1] "What Is Inguinal Hernia ? Information Clearinghouse (NDDIC)." *Inguinal Hernia.* NIDDK, NIH / Michael G. Sarr, M.D., Mayo Clinic, Dec. 2008. Web. 2012.

Hydroceles

Notice the men pictured in the bottom row on pages 30-31. In addition to the bulge in their groin, each has a swollen scrotum caused by a hydrocele. A hydrocele (HI-droe-seal) is a fluid-filled sac surrounding a testicle that results in swelling of the scrotum. Older boys and adult men can develop a hydrocele due to inflammation or injury within the scrotum. Inflammation may be the result of a testicular infection. Usually the only indication of a hydrocele is a painless swelling of one or both testicles. Adult men with a hydrocele may experience discomfort from the heaviness of a swollen scrotum. Sometimes, the swollen testicle may be smaller in the morning and larger later in the day.

A hydrocele requires treatment if it gets large enough to cause discomfort or disfigurement. Treatment approaches includes surgical excision or needle aspiration.

Removal of a hydrocele may be performed on an outpatient basis using general or spinal anesthesia. The surgeon may make an incision in the scrotum or lower abdomen to remove the hydrocele. If a hydrocele is discovered during surgery to repair an inguinal hernia, a doctor may remove it even if it's causing no discomfort.

Needle aspiration is another option is to remove the fluid in the scrotum with a needle. The injection of a thickening or hardening (sclerosing) drug after the aspiration may help prevent the fluid from reaccumulating.

Aspiration and injection may be an option for men who have risk factors that make surgery more dangerous.[2]

[2] Staff, Mayo Clinic. "Hydrocele." *Mayo Clinic.* Mayo Foundation for Medical Education and Research, 03 Nov. 2011. Web. 2012.

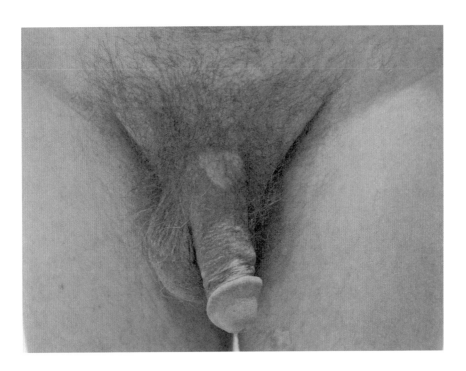

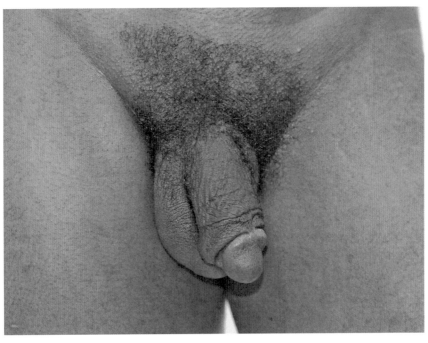

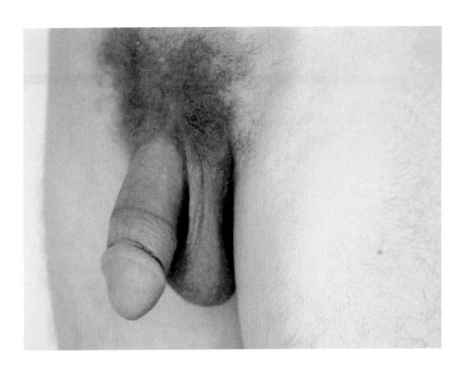

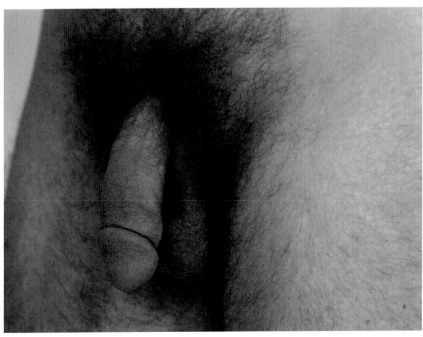

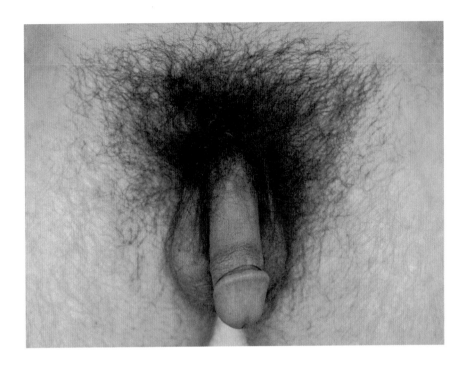

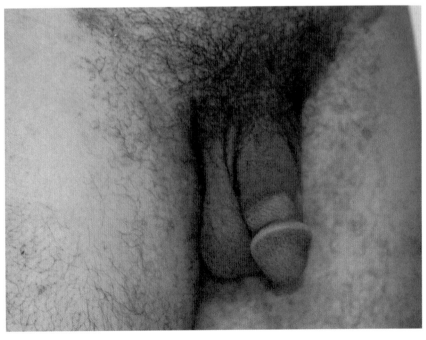

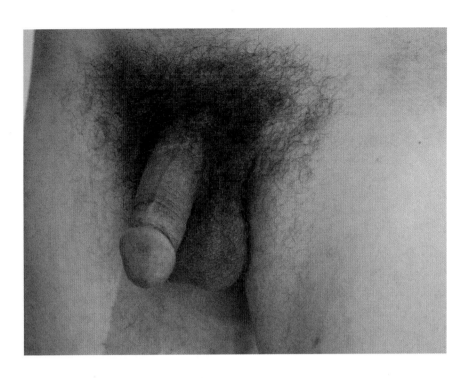

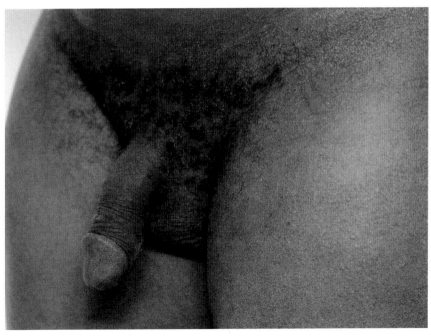

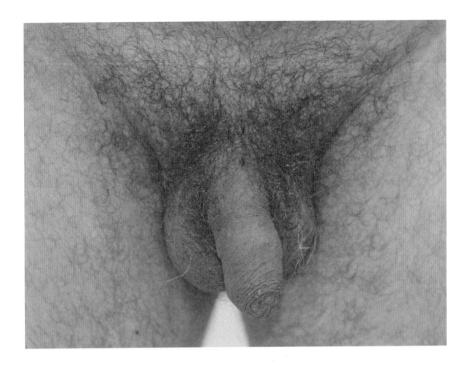

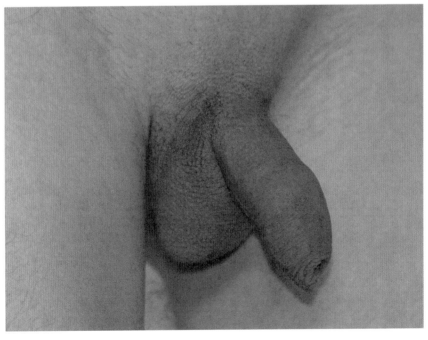

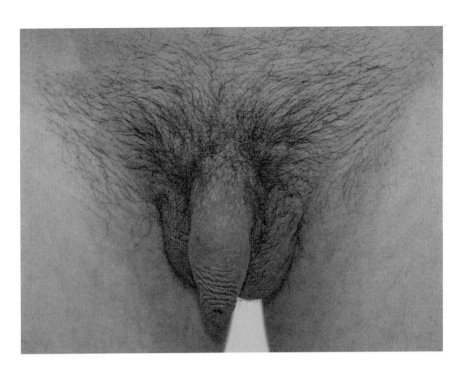

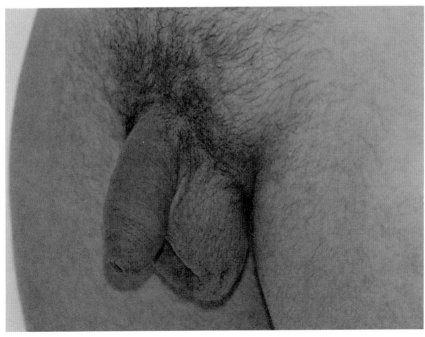

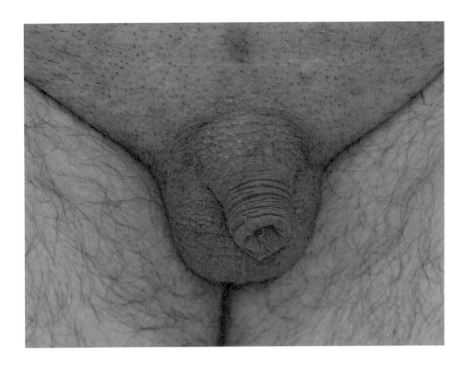

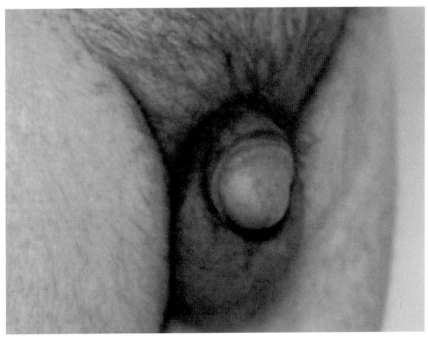

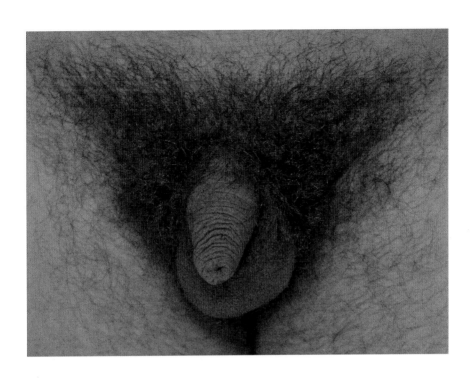

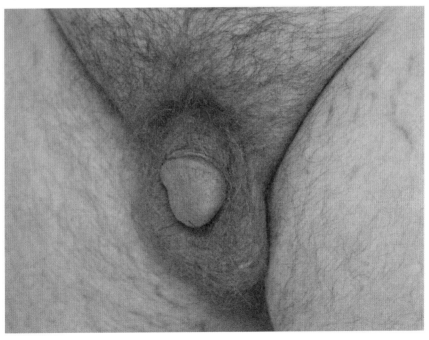

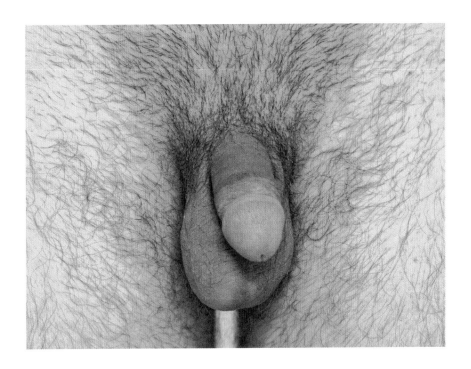

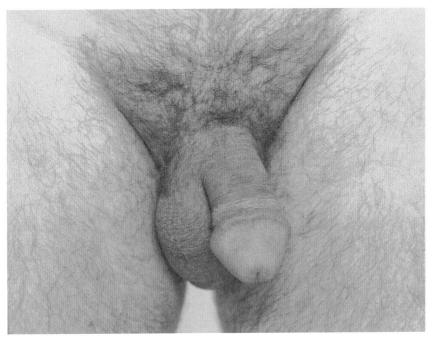

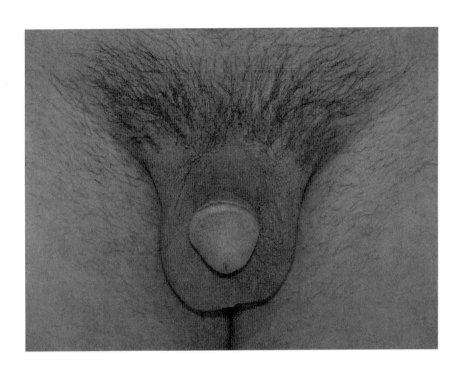

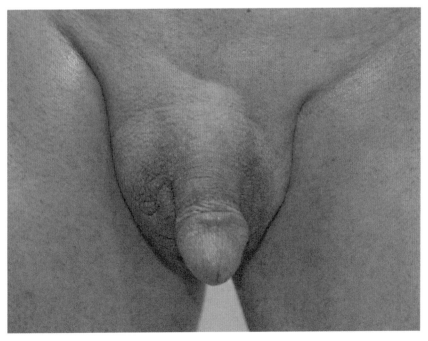

The Men: Exposed continued

One quiet morning, a young man walked in looking like he stepped out of a romance novel. He had lightly tanned skin, short dark hair, and light eyes – even clothed, you could tell his body looked carved from stone. I couldn't put my finger on his ethnicity and that made him even more attractive. He was every woman's man. He claimed he was ex-military and currently a student who was working his way through school on a VA loan and fees from his personal training business. It was abundantly clear he knew he was on top of the hottie chart. When the shoot started, he commented to me that his "package" must be the best I had seen yet. I laughingly told him that was privileged information. After he left, I opened a couple of windows to cool myself off, and then called a couple of my very close girlfriends to tell them about this guy. What a moment! Truth be told, though his package was special indeed, it was not the crown jewel of my project.

Among my clientele were a number of men who worked as "life figure models." The first person I photographed from this field was 50ish and gave me the distinct impression that he did the modeling work to fulfill some sort of fetish. He informed me multiple times that he was comfortable being photographed with an erection, as long as I was okay with him masturbating to keep it in that state. I declined.

There was the community college hot shot snickering with his friends about whether or not they should be "hard" for the shoot. The mom inside me was shaking her head wondering when they would grow up; the professional in me told them whatever state their penis happened to be in while I was taking the photos was fine for the purposes of my project. He tried to hustle me for a cut of my business if he brought in more students. I declined.

In response to my ad, many potential models would include a photograph. I opened one man's email to a photo of his nude body reclining on a pillow-puffed bed. He was bald with a flowing, pointy, white beard and had a tapestry of colorful tattoos adorning his tanned, muscular body. He was a charming client, and days later sent me a thank-you email offering to return for a second photo shoot if he could pose along with another man. I sent my regrets.

As word spread through the Life Model Guild that mine was a legitimate and "noble" project, more professional life figure models made appointments to participate in my research. One such man strode in like he owned the world. His towering height, dress, and demeanor gave me the impression that he could have been a tribal chief from a different era. He didn't need small talk, nor a dressing room – just took off his clothes, laid them over a bench, walked to the mark taped on the floor, and struck a pose. Not an elaborate pose, mind you, but anyone would have been impressed. Upon finishing the session, he complimented me on my professionalism and assured me he would spread the word and send more candidates my way. Thank you, client "X."

There was a middle-aged man who was a member of a local nudist community. Though I have lived in this area for more than 20 years, I had no idea that there were a handful of such communities throughout this major metropolitan region. He shared how liberating it was just to be part of the natural surroundings. I later discovered that the overwhelming population in these nudist communities is middle-aged men. Hmmm...

A couple of potential clients came in under the influence. Two were peacefully escorted out. I realized another was high when I received a skanky email proposition from him after he left. More interesting than his request was that though he was only 30ish, it appeared that his testicle(s) were missing given that his scrotum looked like a deflated balloon.

A foreign university student in his early twenties came in. He had recently been offered a modeling job for a fashion show – at 6'1", 165 pounds he was told he was the perfect size for fashion advertising. His motivation for participating in my project was to prove to himself that he could overcome the strict cultural boundaries he had grown up with that pertained to one's body. And he did.

Two elderly men arrived late one morning. One claimed to be the other's caretaker because his friend suffered from Parkinson's disease. They were great. On their way out, one man slapped the other on the back and said: "Hey! We're models! Scratch that off your bucket list." His friend's response: "Not just any models, we're nude models!"

Post Script: A few months later, the romance–novel guy walked into the Starbucks where I was enjoying lattes with my girlfriend. And yes, my heart started racing – as did hers! Though I saw him, no eye contact was made, so I do not know if he saw or even recognized me. There was a collective sigh by all the school drop-off moms as they watched him walk out.

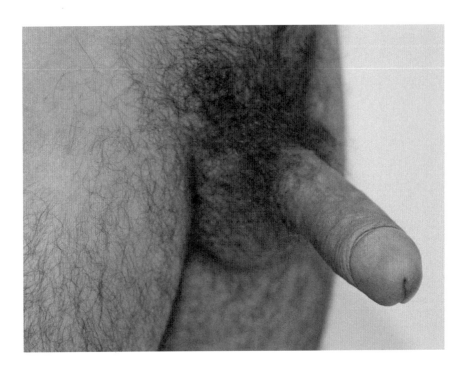

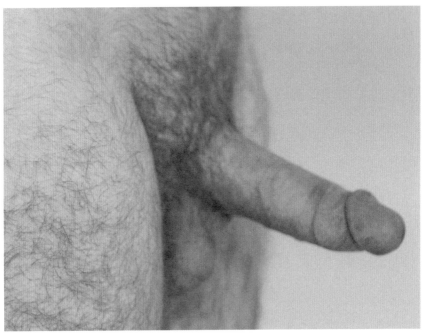

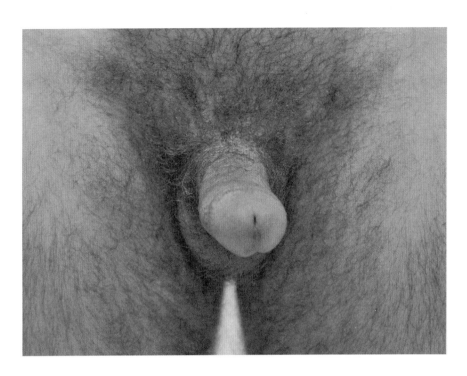

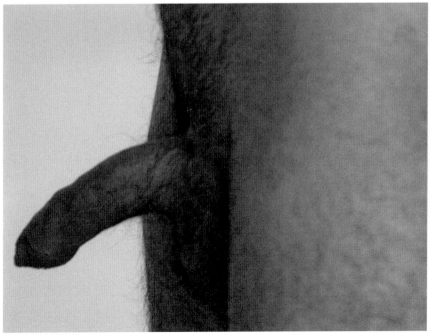

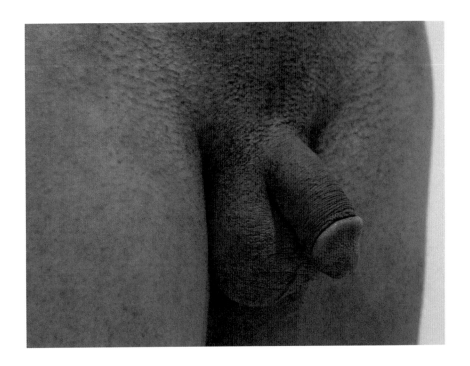

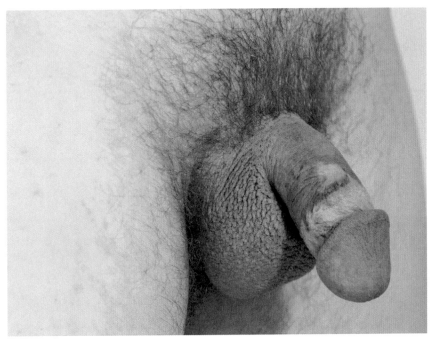

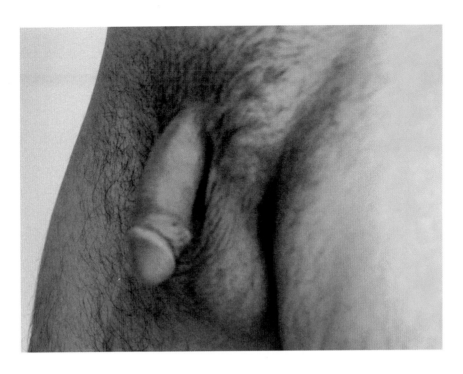

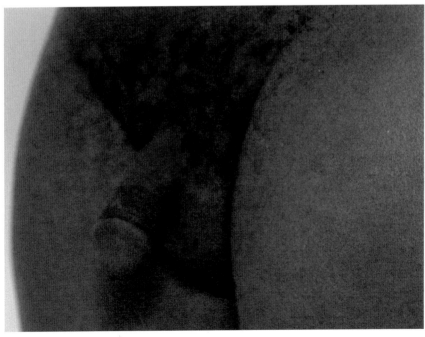

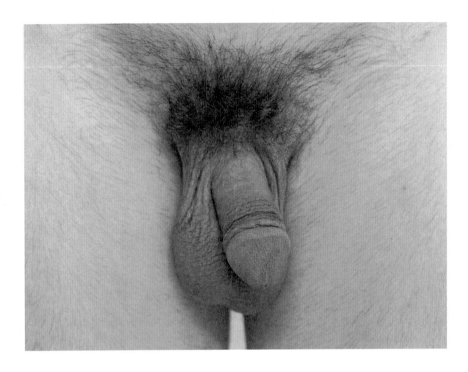

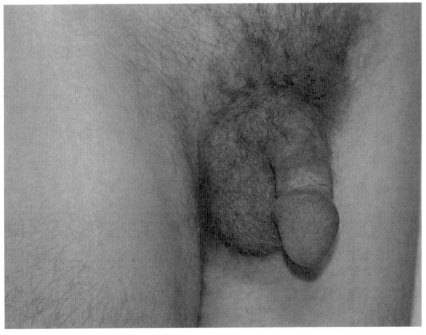

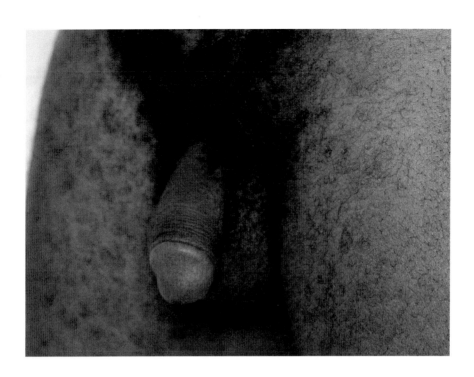

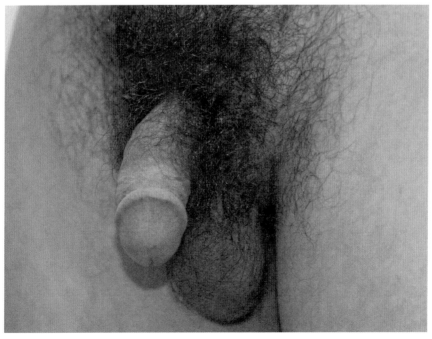

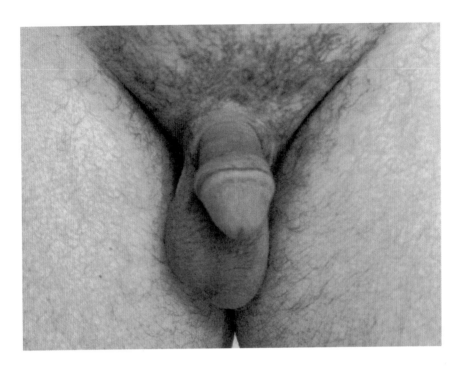

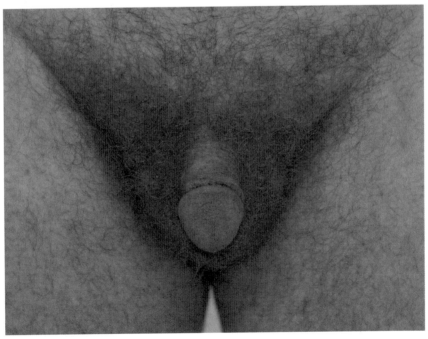

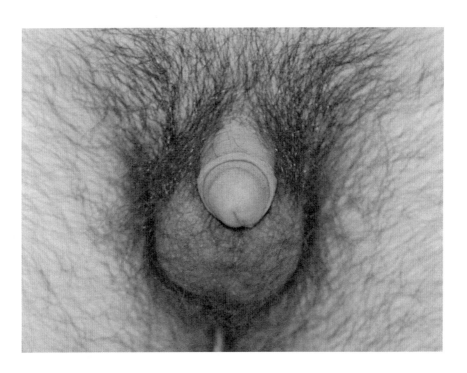

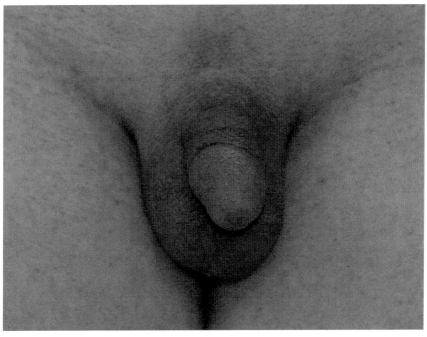

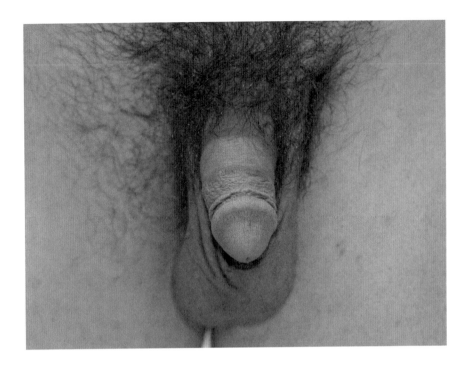

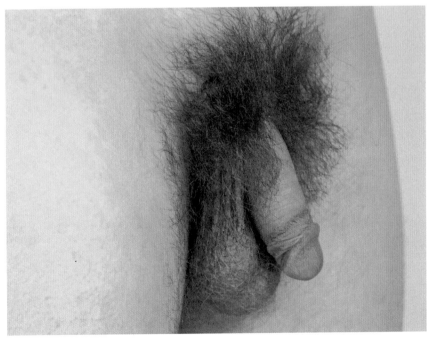

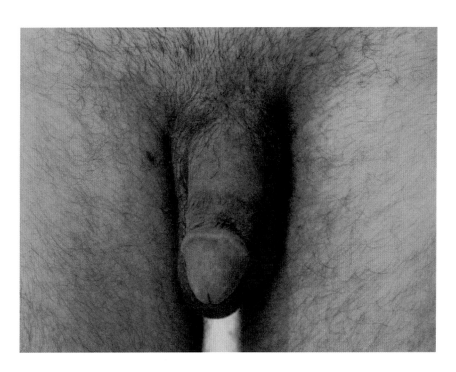

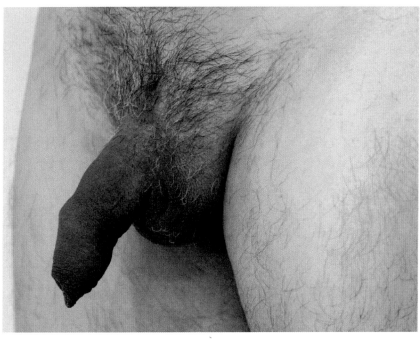

Circumcision

Support of Circumcision

Circumcision is practiced for religious, cultural, social, and healthcare reasons. There is conclusive evidence from worldwide observational and medical studies that circumcised men have a significantly lower risk of sexually transmitted diseases, includ-ing HIV/AIDS.

Approximately 34% of males worldwide are circumcised, of whom two-thirds are estimated to be Muslim.[1,2] Circumcising newborn boys is a common practice in Israel (92%), much of the Middle East (91%), the United States (79%), and Australia (59%); less so in Canada (44%), Central Asia, and Africa. There is increasing demand for safe, low-cost, male circumcision in southern Africa as a protection against the spread of HIV.[3]

History of Circumcision

Genesis 16-21: "...And God said unto Abraham, 'Thou shalt keep my covenant therefore, thou, and thy seed after thee in their generations. This is my covenant, which ye shall keep, between me and you and thy seed after thee. Every man-child among you shall be circumcised. And ye shall circumcise the flesh of your foreskin; and it shall be a token of the covenant betwixt me and you'".

This was not the beginning of circumcision in the world; it was simply the introduction of a well-known practice, already common among Egyptians and others, to Abraham's family and descendants.[4]

Today, Muslims are the largest religious group to circumcise their male offspring. This ritual shows belonging and closeness to their spiritual ancestor and physical forefather, the Prophet Ibrahim.

The Holy Qur'an 16:123: "Then We inspired you: 'Follow the religion of Ibrahim, the upright in Faith'". And part of the religion of Ibrahim is circumcision. Circumcision was practiced by all Muslim prophets hence, and historically established as an Islamic ritual.

Unlike the Jewish tradition, circumcision in Islam is not a symbol of Allah's covenant with humans. The prophet Mohammed is reported to have stated, "Circumcision is *sunnah* (customary or traditional) for the men."[5] Besides submission to the Will of God, male circumcision is an important tradition aimed at improving hygiene. Therefore, in Arabic, circumcision is also known as *tahara*, meaning purification or cleanliness.[5]

Opposition to Circumcision

The development of the prepuce (foreskin) is incomplete in the newborn male child, and separation from the glans (penis head), rendering it retractable, does not usually occur until some time between nine months and three years. During the first year or two of life, when the infant is incontinent, the prepuce fulfills an essential function in protecting the glans.

There are many and varied reasons for circumcising infants. None are convincing to the opponents of the practice. Though early circumcision is said to prevent penile cancer, good hygiene to keep the prepuce clean would have a like effect in preventing this disease.

Douglas Gairdner, D.M., M.R.C.P., Consultant Pediatrician, United Cambridge Hospitals in Volume 2 of the 1949 British Medical Journal reported: "In the light of these facts a conservative attitude towards the prepuce is proposed, and a routine for its hygiene is suggested. If adopted this would eliminate the vast majority of the tens of thousands of circumcision operations performed annually in this country."[6] Great Britain adopted his recommendation; and, in the decade that followed, recouped millions of pounds in related medical expenses.

American Academy of Pediatrics Position Statement Existing scientific evidence demonstrates potential medical benefits of newborn male circumcision; however, the data is not sufficent to recommend routine neonatal circumcision. In circumstances where there are potential benefits and risks, yet the procedure is not essential to the child's current well being, parents should determine what is in the best interest of the child. To make an informed choice, parents of all male infants should be given accurate and unbiased information and be provided the opportunity to discuss this decision. If a decision for circumcision is made, procedural analgesia should be provided.[7]

[1]Waskett, Jake H. "Circumcision Independent Reference and Commentary Service." Global Circumcision Rates. CIRCS.org, 25Apr.2012

[2] "Abraham and Origins of Jewish Circumcision." *Aboutcirc.com*. N.p. 2005

[3] "Male Circumcision: Global Trends and Determinants of Prevalence, Safety and Acceptability." *World Health Organization*. World Health Organization, 14 Dec. 2007. Web. 2012.

[4] "Male Circumcision - the Islamic View." Converting to Islam. N.p., 2009.

[5] "Circumcision of Boys." *BBC News*. BBC, 13 Aug. 2009. Web. 2012.

[6] BRITISH MEDICAL JOURNAL, Volume 2, Number 4642: Pages 1433-1437, The Fate of The Foreskin: A Study of Circumcision by Douglas Gairdner, D.M., M.R.C.P., Consultant Paediatrician, United Cambridge Hospitals, December 24, 1949. Web. 2012

[7] American Academy of Pediatrics: Circumcision Policy Statement *Pediatrics AAP Policy. N.p., 27 . peds.2012-1989. Web. 2012*

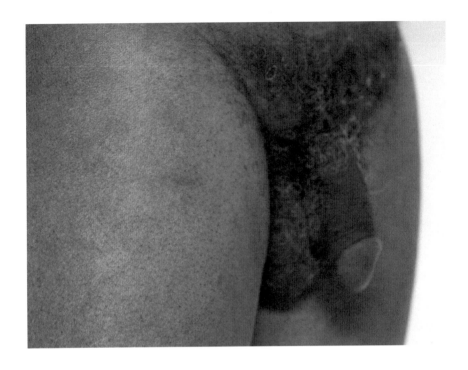

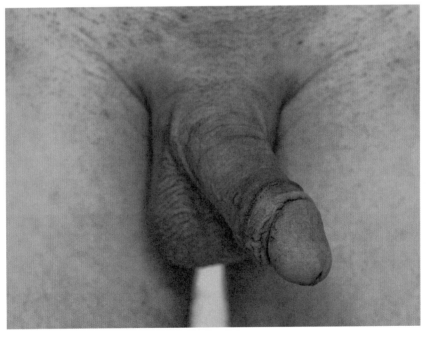

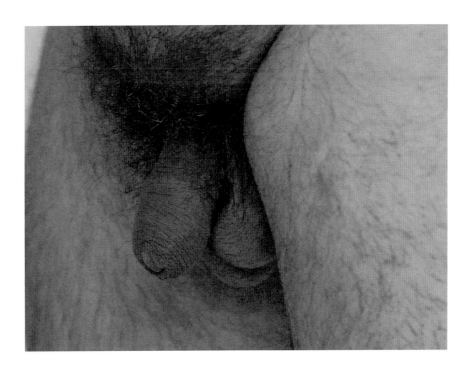

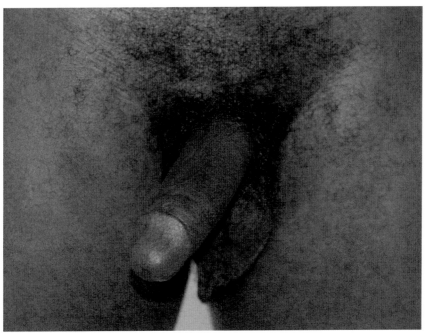

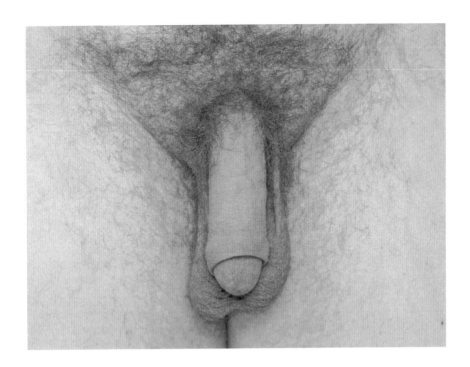

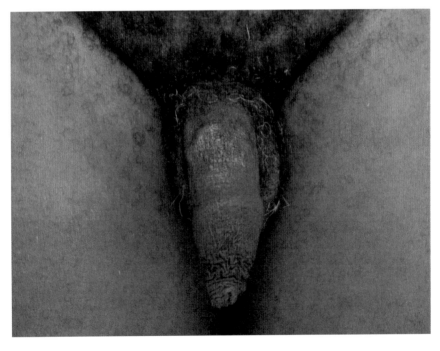

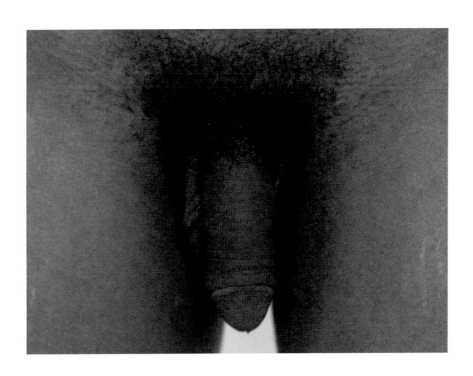

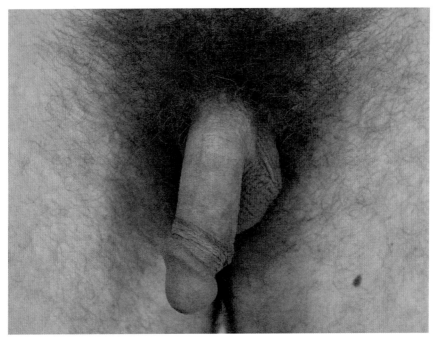

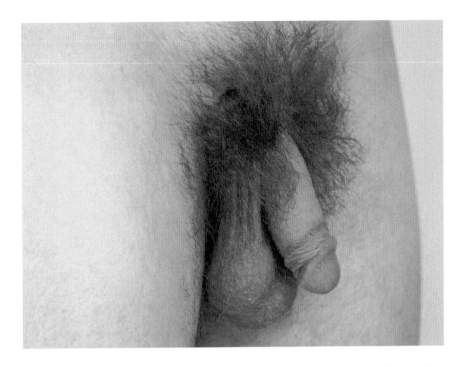

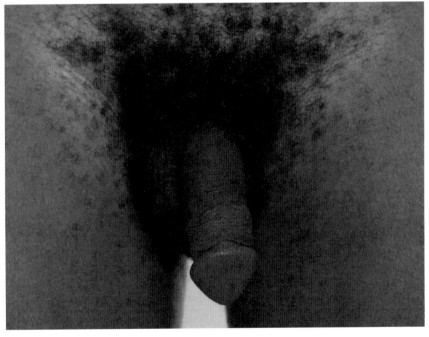

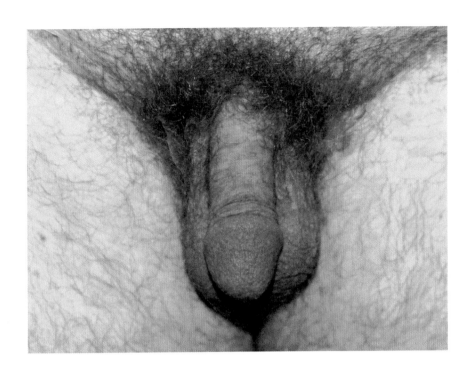

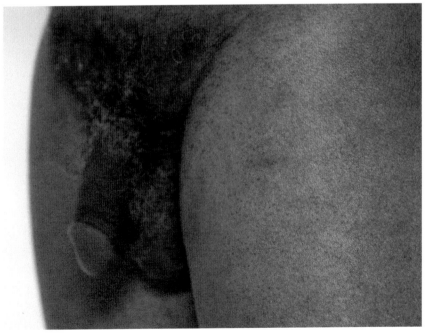

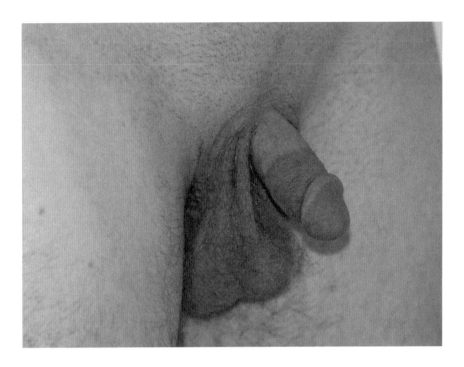

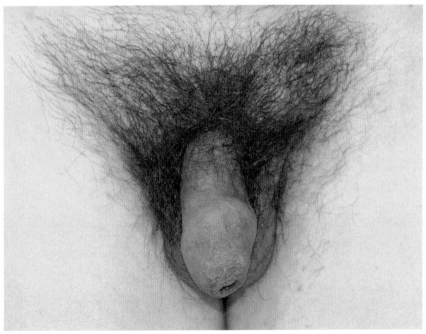

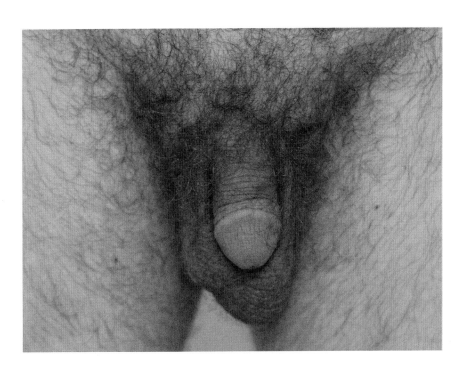

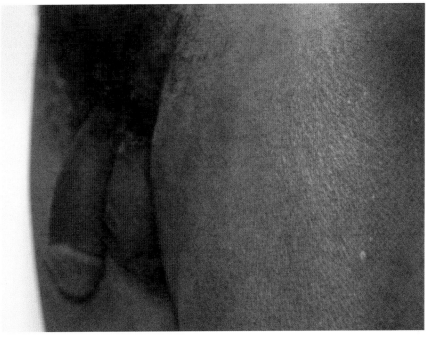

Believe It Or Not

Diphallia (also known as penile duplication) is a condition in which a male is born with two penises, oftentimes along with other genitourinary or gastrointestinal defects. Sufferers are at a higher risk of spina bifida than men with one penis. It is a rare disorder with only 1,000 cases recorded. One in 5.5 million men in the United States has two penises.

Characteristics of Diphallia

Those in possession of a diphallus tend to be sterile, due to either congenital defects or difficulties in application. Urine and semen may be passed by both penises, by only one, or through some other aperture in the perineum.

A range of duplication types have been seen, from organs that fissure into two, to the presence of two distinct penises positioned at some distance from each other. Most diphalluses lie side by side and are of equal size, but they also can be seated atop one another, with one distinctly larger than the other.

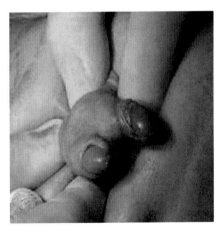

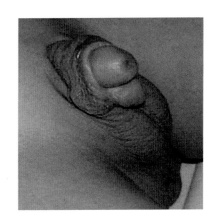 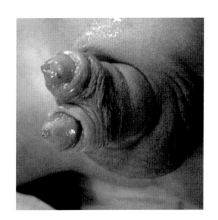

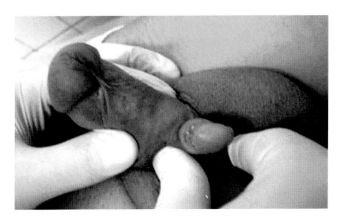

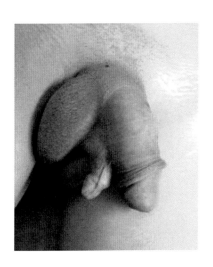 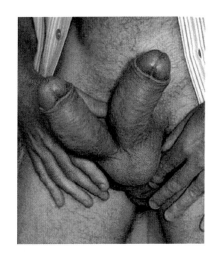

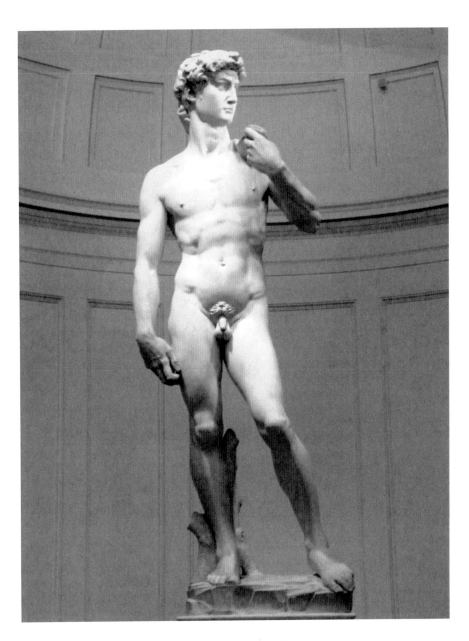

Michelangelo's David

Galleriae dell'Accademia in Florence, Italy

Afterword

The Private Square: Penises was written because heretofore there has been no place for people to see a non-retouched, non-pornographic sampling of real-life penises. As my idea blossomed into production, I decided to expand *The Private Square* into a series of books to showcase the sexual anatomy of both men and women. Being dissatisfied with one's body is a ubiquitous concern among adolescents and many adults in the United States and other size-conscious countries. My objective for *The Private Square* changed from a desire to appease curiosity to a means by which everyone could see that his or her body parts were normal, albeit different.

The Private Square series: *Volume 1: Penises, Volume 2: Breasts, Vol-ume 3: Vulvas,* and *Volume 4: Buttocks* addresses those concerns by showing hundreds of actual photos depicting the sexual anatomy of multi-cultural people aged 18 to 80. *The Private Square* shows each of us that there is an amazing range of normality, in hopes of encouraging people to accept and love their body. Confidence in oneself translates to greater mental health and happiness. By feeling that our body is normal and accepting the way we look, we take an incredible step forward to a positive body image. Within the pages of this series you shall see that everyone fits in.

The Private Square encourages us to regard our body as a gift. So for you, your sons', daughters' and friends' sake, share this book and make someone's day.

We all have good bodies – they're just unique ones.

Made in the USA
Las Vegas, NV
04 June 2023

72973332R00055